REVITALIZE & RENEW

Jennifer Khosla

Bill –
Live well!

REVITALIZE & RENEW

7 DAYS TO A HEALTHIER YOU

Jennifer Khosla

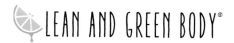 LEAN AND GREEN BODY®

Photography by Lauren Rossi & Nik Wilcox

CreateSpace, Charleston, SC.
Available from Amazon.com, CreateSpace.com, and other retail outlets.

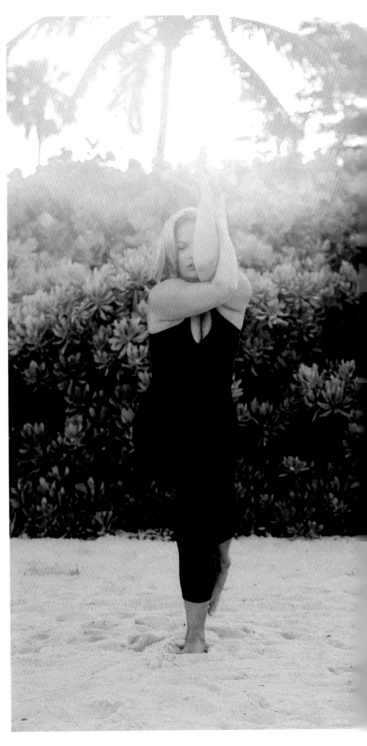

DISCLAIMER

In consideration of beginning a detox program, I the reader, do herby waive, release, and forever discharge Lean and Green Body® / Jennifer Khosla, and all other from any and all responsibility or liability for injuries, illnesses or damages resulting from my participation in this process. All information provided is property of Lean and Green Body® / Jennifer Khosla, and is not to be used for any other purpose. The information provided is to be used as a guideline.

Keep in mind that any detoxification program may make you feel weak, tired, and irritable, and may cause headaches, dizziness, upset stomach, nausea, weight loss, and diarrhea. While these symptoms can be part of the detoxification process, always check with a qualified health care provider before beginning.

I, the reader, do hereby further acknowledge that I have either had a physical examination and have been given a physician's permission to participate or that I have decided to participate in the detox program without the approval of my physician and do hereby assume all responsibility. I, the reader, accept the above agreement of release of liability and terms of this disclaimer and I, the reader, assume full responsibility.

No book can replace the care and service of a trained doctor, you should always consult with your physician for questions related to your health.

Following the detox and tips recommended in this book does not ensure that you will be healthy. Your health is the result of many factors, it is important that you rely on the advice of a health care professional for your specific situation and needs.

We have made every effort to present this information as clear and accurate as possible; however not every situation can be anticipated, and the information presented does not take the place of working with a trained doctor.

TABLE OF CONTENTS

ABOUT THE AUTHOR

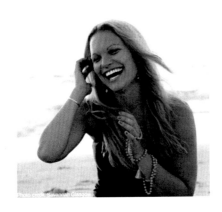

Jennifer Khosla is the founder and CEO of Lean and Green Body®, located in Naples, Florida. Jennifer is a Mind Body Wellness Practitioner and a Holistic Nutrition Specialist.

A wellness expert, she has been working in the fitness and nutrition industry for over a decade. She specializes in Holistic Nutrition, Yoga, and Personal Training.

Jennifer's ability to see each client, and each individual body, as unique is what has made her company stand out. Jennifer started Lean and Green Body® in 2013, and now leads a team of professionals in Southwest Florida.

Jennifer wrote this book based off her popular detox workshops in Naples. This book is an opportunity for Jennifer to share her knowledge, passion, and excitement for nutrition and full body wellness with those around the world.

Her drive and fearless personality has allowed her to grow Lean and Green Body® into what it is today. Thanks to technology, Jennifer sees clients nationally, monitors their progress, and trains them while they travel. This is only the beginning for Jennifer and Lean and Green Body®.

INTRODUCTION

REVITALIZE & RENEW:
7 DAYS TO A HEALTHIER YOU!

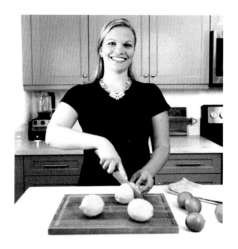

Complete with over 13 recipes and a detailed explanation on easing in and out of your cleanse. This book is loaded with tips and recipes to guide you to a healthier lifestyle once you have completed the detox. You'll learn the benefits of cleansing, how to cleanse, and the many physical and mental benefits of cleansing.

I created this cleanse as a way to make detoxing (or cleansing) our bodies more accessible to everyone. I have expanded upon our original detox and provided additional insights about the cleansing process. Most detox guides are loaded with high sugar concoctions and do not provide nearly enough nutrients for your body to sustain. This book provides guidelines on how to prepare for and execute the detox, which will maximize nutrient absorption in the body, allowing you to feel your best. I will guide you through the entire process of the detox, and provide you with step by step instruction for creating healthy habits post detox. After completing the detox, you will be able to create and sustain a healthy lifestyle that meets your specific goals.

WHY DETOX?

Our food, our environment, and our lives (in general) are loaded with so many toxins, heavy metals, and pollutants. There are daily steps that you can take to protect yourself from these dangers, which you'll learn later in this book. It is essential for us to cleanse our bodies and let go of all these toxins in order to live our healthiest lives possible. In my opinion, detoxing is something that should be done regularly, perhaps four times per year. Even the healthiest eaters can use a detox to regulate their system, allow the digestive system time to rest, and let go of any remaining heavy metals, toxins, or pollutants that are acquired through daily life. Personally, I like to cleanse when the seasons change.

Detoxing is a great opportunity to cleanse your body of toxins, heavy metals, excess sugar, excess sodium, and free radicals. We all tend to over indulge every now and then. Our weeks are full, working 10+ hours a day at our jobs, and then we have the responsibility of taking care of our family, children, pets, and the house. It often seems like there are not enough hours in the day to get everything accomplished. When the weekend arrives, we feel free! We use these two weekend days to experience as much freedom and relaxation as we can. Often times straying from our diet, we binge on foods that we know will not provide any substantial nutrients for the body. Many clients ask me if they can have a "cheat" day at least once during the week. I typically reply, "no". If we cheated, and strayed from our meal plan every weekend, that is approximately 104 days your body is working overtime to remove the junk from your body. That number is astounding. Instead of looking for ways to cheat yourself, look for ways in which you can help propel yourself forward.

"When doing a detox, it is important to rest the gastrointestinal system, mainly because it works so hard at digesting processed, rich fatty foods, and chemicals daily."

Detoxing can go very wrong when it is taken to the extreme. While I understand the need for some individuals to do the 'Master Cleanse' and survive off water, lemon, cayenne pepper, and maple syrup, for spiritual or dietary needs - I feel that this is not a fit for most people. This type of detox cleanses your body from any food remaining in your digestive system, and allows your gastrointestinal system time to rest and perhaps heal. However while on this cleanse, you are consuming virtually no calories. The main source of your calories is from maple syrup…sugar. There is only so much sugar that our bodies can handle before it is stored in our fat cells. **When doing a detox, it is important to rest the gastrointestinal system, mainly because it works so hard at digesting processed, rich fatty foods, and chemicals daily.** Processed food and chemicals are very tough on our bodies. Our bodies are designed to digest pure food in its natural state. It is just as important to flood your body with nutrients. This is accomplished by drinking juices and smoothies, which provides your body with nutrients, essential vitamins, minerals, and enzymes. Even though you are not consuming the standard three square meals per day, you are still receiving the nutrients your body requires.

WHAT YOU CAN EXPECT FROM YOUR DETOX

When detoxing, you will begin to experience many changes in your body, not just physical changes. You will notice a clearer, more focused mind and an increase in energy. You may experience better digestion, less bloating, gas, and digestive upset. Detoxing can help to reduce inflammation in the body, especially inflammation in the skeletal and digestive systems. You may notice clearer skin, better quality of sleep, and an improved and more positive mood. Detoxing may help to jumpstart your weight loss journey, which will inevitably improve your overall health.

EASING INTO YOUR DETOX

Easing into your detox is an exciting time! Perhaps this is your first detox, and you are unsure what to expect. Or maybe you are a regular detoxer and are ready to get this detox started! No matter your experience, this is the perfect detox for almost anyone.

This detox is specifically designed to help you cleanse out heavy metals, detox your liver and kidneys, and rest your gastrointestinal system. Our digestive system works so hard breaking down, digesting, and eliminating our food daily. Our food supply is polluted with chemicals, pesticides, and genetically modified organisms (GMO's); the food we eat is no longer pure and naturally organic. Our body has trouble recognizing these chemicals and breaking them down, which ultimately wreaks havoc on our bodies.

When we eat real food, organic pure food that is bioavailable, our bodies are able to recognize this food. It is able to more efficiently break it down and utilize the nutrients efficiently, and eliminate what we no longer need. *Our goal should be to consume organic bioavailable food daily!* However, sometimes we overindulge (life happens!), and now we need to reset. This is where detoxing comes into play.

"Our goal should be to consume organic bioavailable food daily!"

What's the difference between cleansing and detoxing?
Is there really a difference between cleansing and detoxing? Not exactly as these terms are often interchangeable. Cleansing and detoxing are both tools to clean out our bodies of toxins, heavy metals, pollutants, and inflammation. Cleansing and detoxing allows us to let go of any excess chemicals, sugars, sodium, unhealthy eating habits, and anything that we may be holding onto that we no longer need, both physically and mentally. This allows us to be lighter, lifted, and open to a healthier way of living.

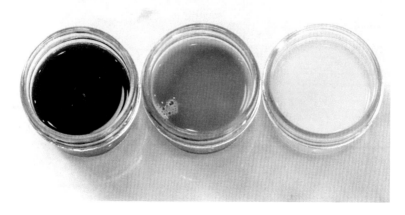

What's the difference between juices and smoothies?

This detox utilizes juices, smoothies and solid food recipes to make the detox more achievable and easier on the psyche. Juicing is wonderful and very alkalizing for the body. There is virtually no fiber in juice, making it easy for our body to breakdown, utilize the nutrients, and excrete what we do not need...very little digestive energy is needed. This is great for someone with leaky gut or a digestive issue. Allowing the digestive system time to rest, heal and recover is crucial. Smoothies, on the other hand, contain the entire fruit or vegetable, including the fiber. Smoothies require more digestive energy and work from our bodies, but provides us with macronutrients (fiber, fat and protein); which are essential to an alkalized and cleansed body!

CLEANSE YOUR BODY FROM THE INSIDE OUT

Some things to consider prior to beginning your detox. First consider, why you are choosing to detox. Are you looking to start a new, healthier lifestyle? Looking to eliminate meat, dairy, gluten, or sugar? Perhaps you are looking to identify a food allergen or intolerance? Do you want to lose a few extra pounds and jumpstart your wellness plan?

Regardless of your reason, congratulations on taking the first step towards a healthier lifestyle. This detox is a wonderful tool that you will be able to use over and over again. Lean and Green Body® recommends that you cleanse and detox your body about four times per year, perhaps as the seasons change. It can also be beneficial to do a short 24 hour cleanse once per month, selecting one day's worth of recipes from our plan.

Cleansing and detoxing your body can bring up many different emotions and feelings as your body undergoes some major renovations. Cleaning up your diet and lifestyle may inspire you to clean up some other areas of your life as well. Perhaps letting go of negativity, letting go of unnecessary baggage or any thoughts that do not serve you. Whatever is holding you back, or holding you down, let it go. Free yourself from those thoughts, ideas, or relationships. Begin to discover your best self. We find journaling to be very helpful and immensely beneficial during a cleanse; allowing you a clear space to understand your thoughts during the process. Cleanse your body from the inside out, not only physically but mentally too.

HOW TO MENTALLY PREPARE FOR THE DETOX

Will you be starving? Will your hangry evil twin come out? Will you be able to continue with your regular workout routine? Will you be fatigued? Will you be running to the bathroom every five minutes, or worse yet, will you be stuck in the bathroom all week? My clients have brought me every fear or anxiety around cleansing, and they are justified fears and concerns. I am here to clear up some misconceptions about the cleansing process. We are looking to re-design the cleansing realm, and create a new approach to detoxing, making detoxing available to everyone.

You will not be starving on this detox. In fact, many of my clients are so full from the amount of liquid, water, tea, juice, and smoothies they consume, many can not even finish the final juice. We strongly suggest that you consume all beverages everyday for the best results.

No need to worry about being hangry during your detox. This detox was designed to keep your energy steady all day, without any major spikes or drops in blood sugar levels due to low glycemic index foods. The recipes have been carefully designed and tested, and includes an abundance of healthy fats, protein, fiber and greens, which will prevent any fatigue and keep you energized.

Depending on your typical workout routine, you may be able to continue your regular workout schedule. However, I often suggest my clients listen to their bodies and see what your body is asking for. Perhaps, instead of hot power yoga everyday, you add in some slow flow with some incredibly cleansing twists.

One of the biggest concerns my clients have with regard to cleansing is bowel movements. Let's take a moment to talk about this "taboo" topic. Everybody poops and that's great! Having a bowel movement is our bodies way of eliminating what it no longer needs. Many people shy away from the conversation about bowel movements, although it is one of the first things I discuss with my nutrition clients. How are your bowel movements? How many times per day do you have a bowel movements? As a Holistic Nutrition Specialist and Mind Body Wellness Practitioner, I always recommend my clients to have a minimum of one substantial bowel movement per day within one hour of waking up, ideally solid. Two to three bowel movements per day would be great, one after every major meal; however our diets, lifestyle, stress, and day to day routines do not always allow for this.

When we are constipated and do not have a bowel movement for 24 hours or more, the toxins from our fecal matter are released back into our bodies. Talk about seriously needing a cleanse! Now take a moment and consider, how are your bowel movements? If you currently are only having one bowel movement per week, then yes you may experience (hopefully!) an increase during this detox. **Side note: if you are only having one bowel movement per week, please consult your Doctor or Nutritionist ASAP!** In all seriousness, you may experience an increase in the number and quality of bowel movements during this detox. This detox is designed to cleanse your body, which can include cleaning out your digestive system.

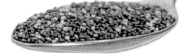

However, please note that if you do not currently drink juices, smoothies, or consume greens daily in your diet, this detox will be an adjustment for your body. You may experience some side effects as your body detoxes and adjusts to this new healthier way of eating. Some possible side effects could include, but are not limited to, diarrhea, nausea, upset stomach, dizziness, headaches, and lightheadedness.

Now let's discuss the detoxification process! Before the actual detox begins, you will want to take a few steps in the days leading up to the detox to prepare your body and mind.

TWO DAYS PRIOR TO THE DETOX, IT IS SUGGESTED THAT YOU ELIMINATE THE FOLLOWING FROM YOUR DIET:

Meat	Added Sugar
Dairy	Added Salt
Soy	Alcohol
Processed Foods	Coffee
Fried Foods	Black Tea

We all have our vices, whether it be coffee, sugar, or alcohol. Regardless of your comfort food, if it is on the list, it has to go during the detox. If you are one of the few who does not believe they have a vice, well you may just learn how much that cup of coffee or glass of wine means to you.

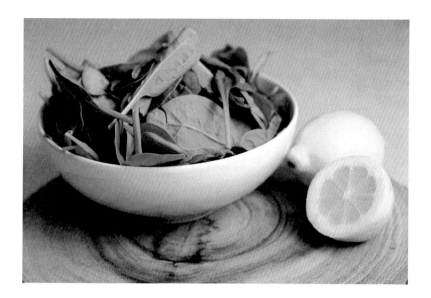

Slowly begin to eliminate these items from your diet. This will prepare you for the cleanse when we begin to eliminate even more and begin resetting the body.

What should you eat two days before the cleanse begins? During this time, focus on plant sources of protein such as legumes, beans, chia seeds, flax seeds, hemp seeds, and nuts. Start adding in a large salad for lunch and/or dinner topped with roasted seasonal vegetables, avocado, and beans. Here are some options leading into the detox.

TRY OUR DETOX APPROVED SUMMER SALAD!

2 cups organic spinach or arugula
1 TBSP extra virgin olive oil
Juice from 1/2 lemon
Sprinkle of pink Himalayan sea salt
1/2 cup black beans

1. Massage spinach or arugula with olive oil, lemon juice, and pink Himalayan sea salt.
2. Top with black beans and one of the vegetable recipes below.

SAUTÉED ZUCCHINI

1 organic zucchini
1 TBSP organic coconut oil

1. Wash zucchini
2. Chop zucchini into small bite size pieces
3. Sauté on medium heat stove top with 1 TBSP of organic coconut oil
4. Stir frequently
5. Cook for 5 minutes or until zucchini softens and browns

SAUTÉED BRUSSELS SPROUTS

1 cup Brussels sprouts
1 TBSP organic coconut oil

1. Wash and trim Brussels sprouts
2. If you did not purchase already shaved Brussels sprouts, then thinly slice your Brussels
3. Add Brussels to stovetop pan, cooking on medium heat with 1 TBSP organic coconut oil
4. Sauté for approximately 5 minutes or until Brussels begin to soften and crisp

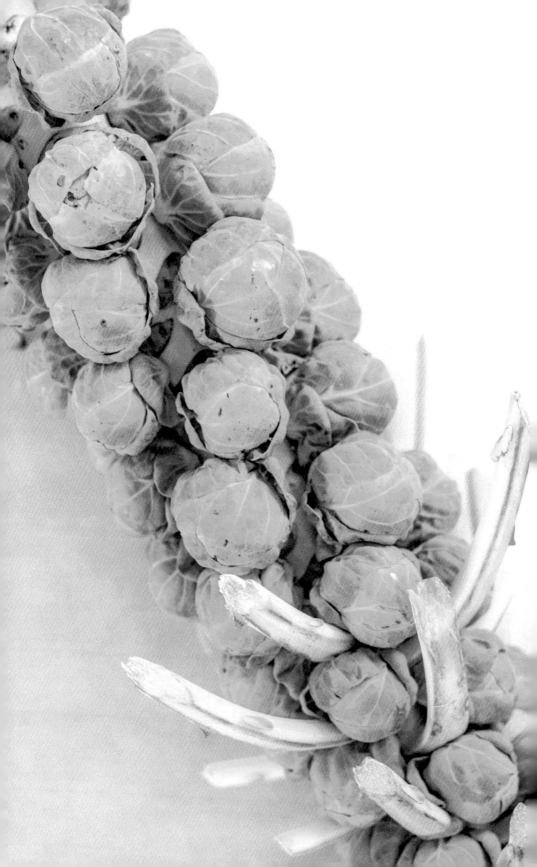

MORNING ROUTINE

Every day on the detox you will begin with my favorite morning routine.

You will continue this daily through the detox and will have the option to incorporate this morning routine post detox into your new healthy lifestyle.

8 oz room temperature water with the juice from 1/2 organic lemon	2 TBSP Bragg's Apple Cider Vinegar with at least 2 oz. water

Our bodies restore, regenerate, and renew while we are sleeping and require hydration immediately upon waking. The room temperature water with organic lemon will help to wake up the body, aid in digestion, stimulate stomach acid and bile production, boost your immune system, and hydrate your body.

Apple Cider Vinegar is one of my favorite 'tricks of the trade' and something I would recommend using daily. I would recommend using a brand of Apple Cider Vinegar such as Bragg's, which is loaded with nutritional benefits. Apple Cider Vinegar has been around for over 1,000 years. This healing tonic helps with everything from skin, giving your skin a youthful and vibrant glow, to regulating calcium metabolism and blood consistency, to relieving women's menstruation symptoms! It even helps to fight viruses, bacteria, and the common cold naturally! One of my favorite benefits of apple cider vinegar is how it aids in digestion and assimilation of our food, and alkalizes our body, making your feel light and full of energy. The Standard American Diet (SAD) is extremely acidic, making it an ideal environment for disease and illness. Adding in more alkalizing foods and apple cider vinegar can help to increase the pH of our bodies, making it an undesirable place for disease and illness.

THROUGHOUT THE DAY

In addition to the morning routine, it is recommended that you drink the following daily.

1. DRINK A MINIMUM OF 64 OUNCES OF PLAIN WATER

Water is essential for the body, and yet many of us go through life perpetually dehydrated. When we are dehydrated it effects all areas of the body. Dehydration prompts our cells to shrink, decreasing athletic performance and causing dizziness, confusion, heart palpitations, fainting, weakness, dry mouth, and an increase in thirst.

It is recommended to drink a minimum of 64 oz of plain water per day, and an additional 8 oz for each cup of caffeine or alcohol you drink.

2. DRINK ONE CUP OF GREEN TEA

Free radicals are highly reactive atoms that have at least one unpaired electron. Electrons like to be paired, so these free radicals look to pair with electrons from other molecules in the body, like your DNA for example. Free radicals can be created within the body or brought in from outside sources, such as smoking, pollution, and other toxins. These free radicals damage our cells, can alter our DNA structure, and can cause cancer. However, the body has a built in defense for these free radicals, called antioxidants. Antioxidants are able to get rid of the free radicals typically before serious damage occurs. Antioxidants can also be found in foods such as goji berries, blueberries, dark chocolate, pecans, artichokes, and many more.

One powerful antioxidant is green tea. Green tea has been around for years, although recently has gained attention again for it's powerful antioxidants. Green tea is packed with polyphenols (flavonoids and catechins) which remove free radicals. These antioxidants protect our body from free radical damage to our cells and help protect us from many diseases and illnesses.

Green tea also contains a compound known as epigallocatechin gallate (EGCG), a potent antioxidant known to help prevent and fight disease, but is popularly known for it's weight loss benefits!

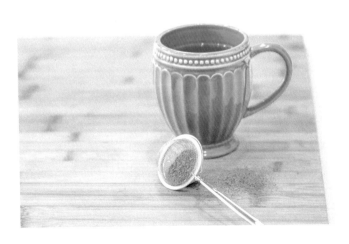

3. DRINK ONE CUP OF PARSLEY TEA

Parsley tea has several benefits and is a great addition to your daily diet. Parsley is loaded with antioxidants and is a natural diuretic, helping to remove free radicals and excess water weight from the body. This tea has been known to aid in healing our digestion system and decreasing inflammation in our body, assisting in the treatment of arthritis, cancer, and other inflammatory conditions.

Please be aware that parsley tea should never be given to a pregnant women since it will stimulate her uterus. Parsley tea is high in oxalic acid and may cause the formation of kidney stones. Parsley tea should not be given to anyone with kidney conditions. As always, please consult your healthcare practitioner if you are unsure if parsley tea is right for you.

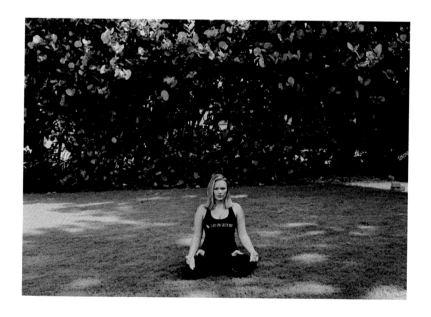

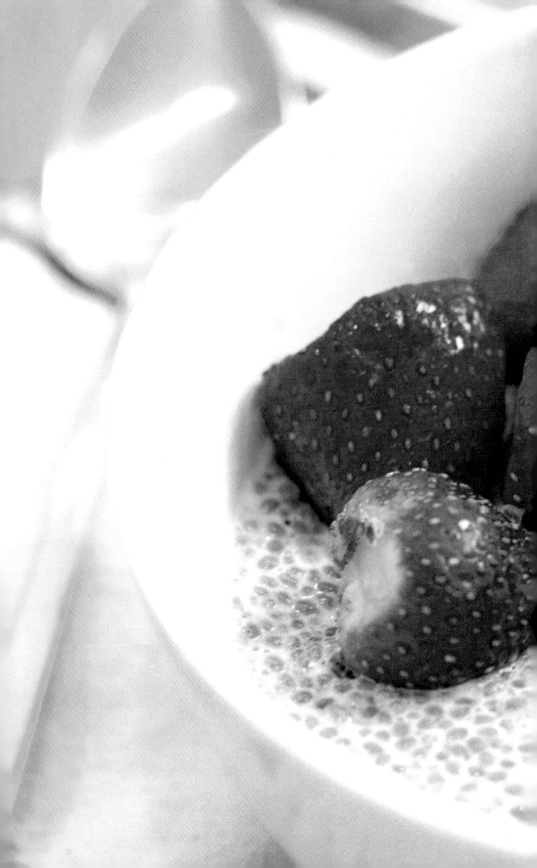

REVITALIZE & RENEW

THE DETOX PLAN

DAY ONE

MORNING

8 oz room temperature water with the juice from 1/2 organic lemon

2 TBSP Bragg's Apple Cider Vinegar with at least 2 oz. water

REMAINDER OF THE DAY

You have five juices to drink today. Spread them out throughout your day, approximately every 2-3 hours.

Drink a minimum of 64 ounces of plain water.

Drink one cup of plain, hot green tea.

Drink one cup of parsley tea.

If you feel faint, dizzy, or lightheaded, have a juice, raw carrots, or watermelon slices.

CONSUME IN THIS ORDER:

1. Blueberry Banana Smoothie   page 71

2. Intoxicating Detoxification Juice   page 53

3. Detox Salad   page 73

4. Grape Citrus Apple Juice   page 57

5. Lean and Green Juice   page 63

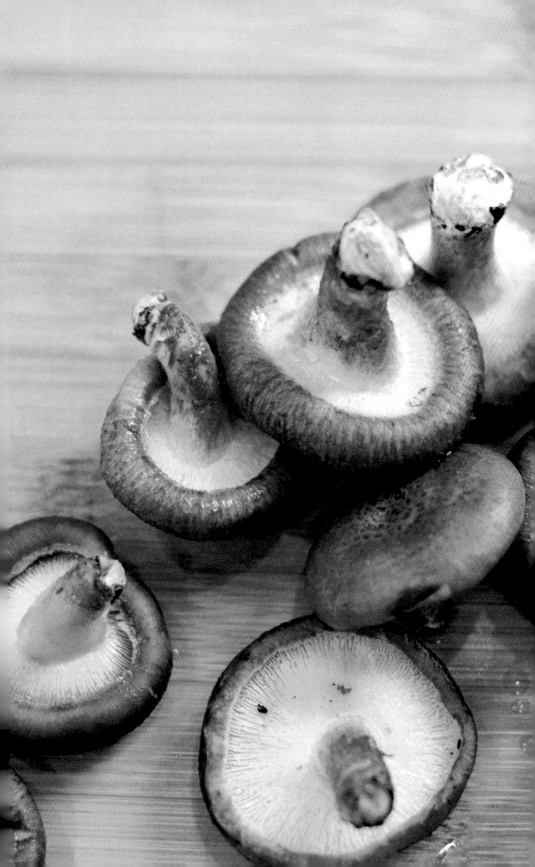

DAY TWO

MORNING

8 oz room temperature
water with the juice from
1/2 organic lemon

2 TBSP Bragg's Apple Cider
Vinegar
with at least 2 oz. water

REMAINDER OF THE DAY

You have five juices to drink today. Spread them out
throughout your day, approximately every 2-3 hours.

Drink a minimum of 64 ounces of plain water.

Drink one cup of plain, hot green tea.

Drink one cup of parsley tea.

If you feel faint, dizzy, or lightheaded, have a juice, raw
carrots, or watermelon slices.

CONSUME IN THIS ORDER:

1. Chia Seed Pudding   page 69

2. Raspberry Lemonade Cleansing Smoothie   page 49

3. Detox Salad   page 73

4. Immunity Juice   page 51

5. Popeye's Blend Juice   page 65

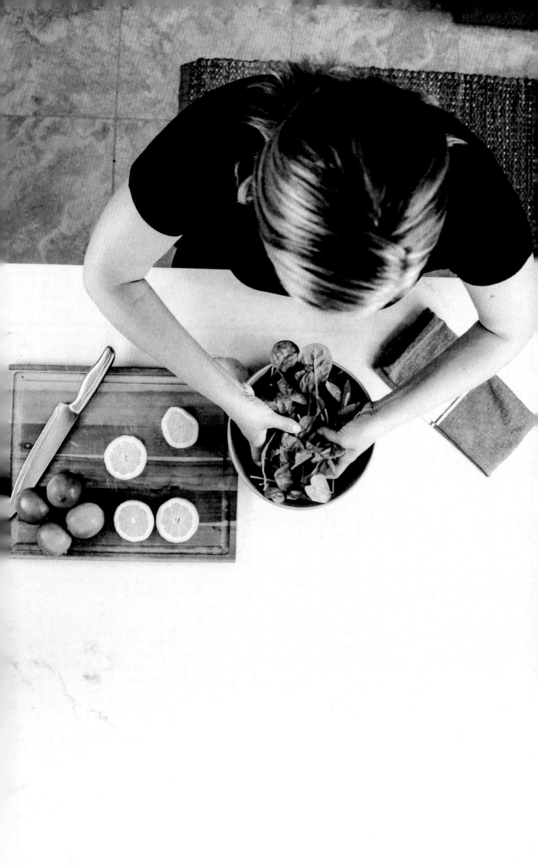

DAY THREE

MORNING

8 oz room temperature water with the juice from 1/2 organic lemon

2 TBSP Bragg's Apple Cider Vinegar with at least 2 oz. water

REMAINDER OF THE DAY

You have five juices to drink today. Spread them out throughout your day, approximately every 2-3 hours.

Drink a minimum of 64 ounces of plain water.

Drink one cup of plain, hot green tea.

Drink one cup of parsley tea.

If you feel faint, dizzy, or lightheaded, have a juice, raw carrots, or watermelon slices.

CONSUME IN THIS ORDER:

1. Raspberry Lemonade Cleansing Smoothie — page 49

2. Green Obsession — page 55

3. Chia Seed Pudding — page 69

4. Orange Carrot Juice — page 67

5. Lean and Green Juice — page 63

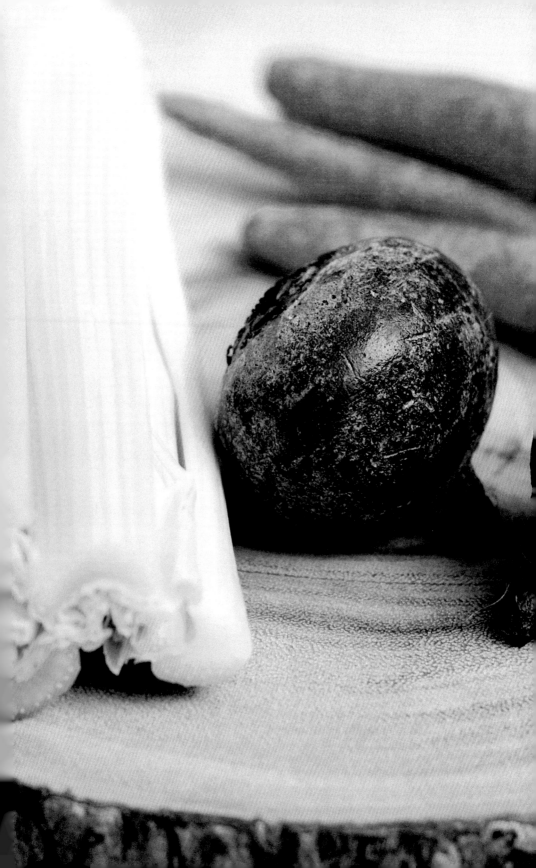

DAY FOUR

MORNING

8 oz room temperature
water with the juice from
1/2 organic lemon

2 TBSP Bragg's Apple Cider
Vinegar
with at least 2 oz. water

REMAINDER OF THE DAY

You have five juices to drink today. Spread them out throughout your day, approximately every 2-3 hours.

Drink a minimum of 64 ounces of plain water.

Drink one cup of plain, hot green tea.

Drink one cup of parsley tea.

If you feel faint, dizzy, or lightheaded, have a juice, raw carrots, or watermelon slices.

CONSUME IN THIS ORDER:

1. Grape Citrus Apple Juice   page 57

2. Queen of Green Juice   page 59

3. Green Obsession   page 55

4. Orange Carrot Juice   page 67

5. Immunity Juice   page 51

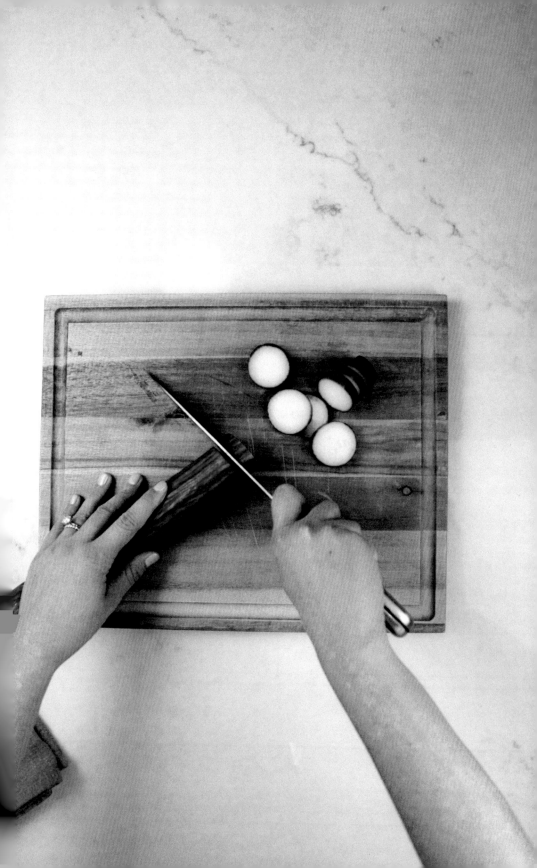

DAY FIVE

MORNING

8 oz room temperature water with the juice from 1/2 organic lemon

2 TBSP Bragg's Apple Cider Vinegar with at least 2 oz. water

REMAINDER OF THE DAY

You have five juices to drink today. Spread them out throughout your day, approximately every 2-3 hours.

Drink a minimum of 64 ounces of plain water.

Drink one cup of plain, hot green tea.

Drink one cup of parsley tea.

If you feel faint, dizzy, or lightheaded, have a juice, raw carrots, or watermelon slices.

CONSUME IN THIS ORDER:

1. Raspberry Lemonade Cleansing Smoothie — page 49

2. Mean Green Juice — page 61

3. Lean and Green Juice — page 63

4. Queen of Green Juice — page 59

5. Intoxicating Detoxification Juice — page 53

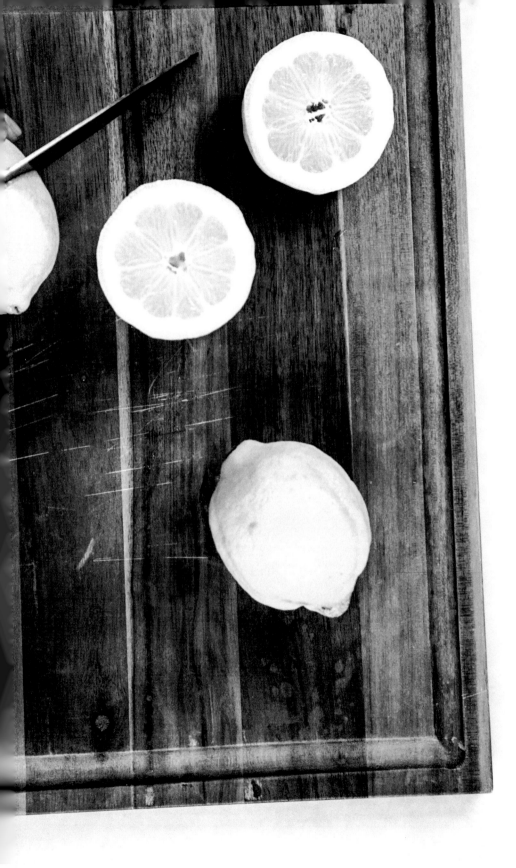

DAY SIX

MORNING

8 oz room temperature
water with the juice from
1/2 organic lemon

2 TBSP Bragg's Apple Cider
Vinegar
with at least 2 oz. water

REMAINDER OF THE DAY

You have five juices to drink today. Spread them out throughout your day, approximately every 2-3 hours.

Drink a minimum of 64 ounces of plain water.

Drink one cup of plain, hot green tea.

Drink one cup of parsley tea.

If you feel faint, dizzy, or lightheaded, have a juice, raw carrots, or watermelon slices.

CONSUME IN THIS ORDER:

1. Immunity Juice   page 51

2. Grape Citrus Apple Juice   page 57

3. Blueberry Banana Smoothie   page 71

4. Popeye's Blend Juice   page 65

5. Green Obsession   page 55

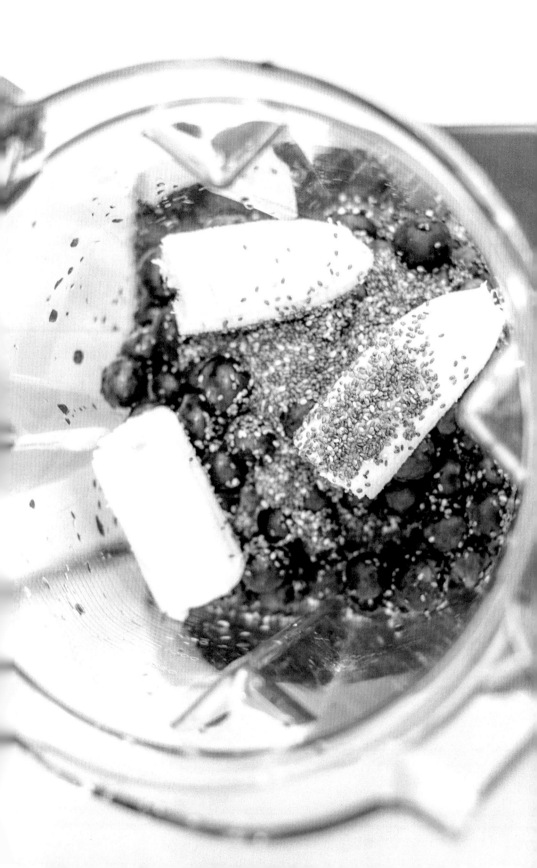

DAY SEVEN

MORNING

8 oz room temperature
water with the juice from
1/2 organic lemon

2 TBSP Bragg's Apple Cider
Vinegar
with at least 2 oz. water

REMAINDER OF THE DAY

You have five juices to drink today. Spread them out throughout your day, approximately every 2-3 hours.

Drink a minimum of 64 ounces of plain water.

Drink one cup of plain, hot green tea.

Drink one cup of parsley tea.

If you feel faint, dizzy, or lightheaded, have a juice, raw carrots, or watermelon slices.

CONSUME IN THIS ORDER:

1. Chia Seed Pudding   page 69

2. Orange Carrot Juice   page 67

3. Detox Salad   page 73

4. Raspberry Lemonade Cleansing Smoothie   page 49

5. Mean Green Juice   page 61

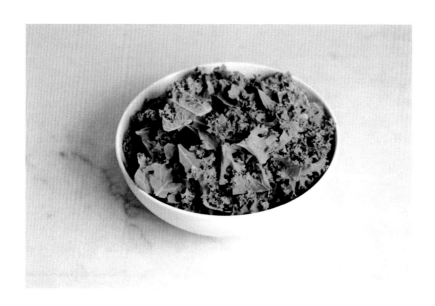

WHILE CLEANSING THE BODY

AVOID:

Meat	Added Sugar
Dairy	Added Salt
Soy	Alcohol
Processed Foods	Coffee
Fried Foods	Black Tea

For optimal results, consume only what is listed for each of the seven days. If you are feeling faint, lightheaded or dizzy, have a snack! Perhaps raw fruit slices or raw vegetables.

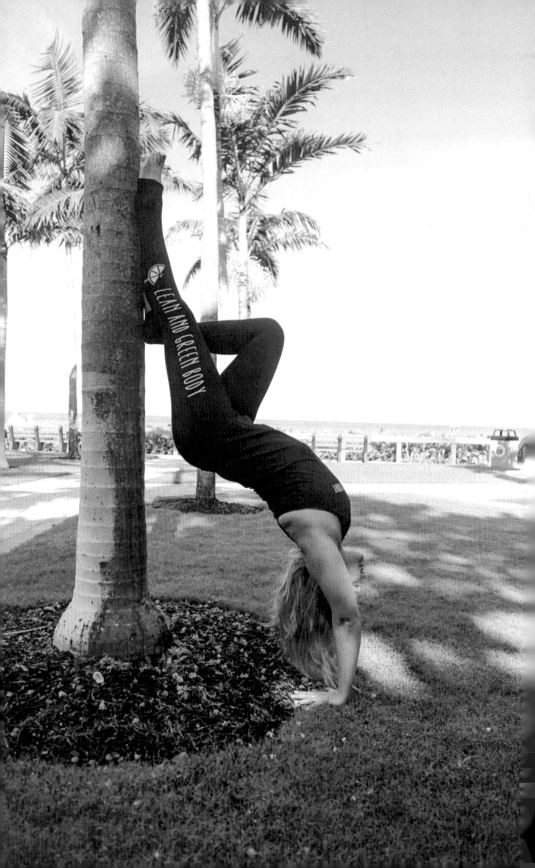

EASING OUT OF YOUR DETOX

Congratulations!! You did it! You have just completed the Lean and Green Body® seven day detox for a healthier you!

You have created an alkaline state for your body, making it an undesirable place for disease and illness. Your body is pure and clean, and you may even consider making some radical changes to your diet as you move forward. Now is the perfect time to try going gluten free, dairy free, vegetarian, or even vegan if you'd like!

As you eat out of your detox, add foods in slowly, listen to your body, see how you feel, and see what your body needs.

Move forward with a more educated awareness of how you fuel your body. Begin to take notice and listen to your body; you'll crave greens and alkaline foods. Take what you have learned over the past seven days and create a healthy new lifestyle.

The first few days out of the cleanse you will want to avoid fatty foods, fried foods, dairy, and anything that is processed. Eating these foods right away may cause serious gastrointestinal upset. Coming out of the cleanse, begin reintroducing foods slowly. This is also a great time to check in for any foods allergies or intolerances. See how your body responds.

Here is an example day for your first few days off the detox.

IDEAL FIRST DAY OUT OF DETOX

Morning Routine (daily)

8 oz room temperature water with 1/2 lemon

1-2 TBSP of apple cider vinegar mixed with at least 2 oz. water

Greens: Choose a green supplement that works for your lifestyle. I am currently loving Garden of Life Raw Organic Perfect Food Greens. I've been using this product for over four years, and it's the only one I serve to my family.

Breakfast

Drink one juice. Perhaps Intoxicating Detoxification

Snack

Almonds. Approximately 23 almonds = 1/4 cup = 1 ounce

Lunch

Drink one juice

Snack

1-2 cups of raw vegetables with 2 TBSP hummus

Dinner

2 cups of fresh, organic arugula massaged with 1/2 lemon, 1 TBSP of extra virgin olive oil, and a sprinkle of sea salt

4-6 oz of lean protein, (fish, chicken, beans, or nuts)

1/2 -1 cup of wild rice or quinoa

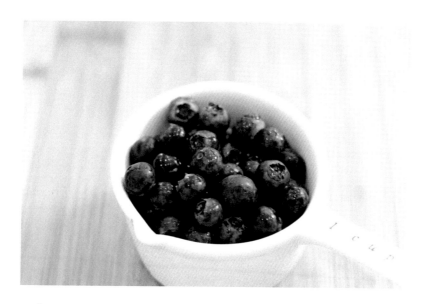

Following this meal plan post detox will help your body adjust to digesting solid food. Introducing one food or food group back into your diet at a time can help you determine food allergies or intolerances. For instance, if you believe you may be sensitive to dairy, try adding one serving of milk or yogurt back into your diet two days post detox. See how your body responds. Any digestive upset? Gas? Bloating? Upset stomach? Eczema? Rash? Hives? Or any other ill side effects? It can be helpful to journal how you feel physically and mentally when adding foods back into your diet. Take note of any physical discomfort, but also notice any brain fog, mood swings, irritability, and fatigue. If you notice any physical or mental side effects from adding dairy, then eliminate it. This is an easy way to decipher what foods your body can and will tolerate, and which foods simply do not suit you. This same pattern can be repeated with any food, but be sure to only test one food at a time.

LEAN AND GREEN BODY®
7 DAY DETOX RECIPES

EACH RECIPE WILL MAKE ONE SERVING.

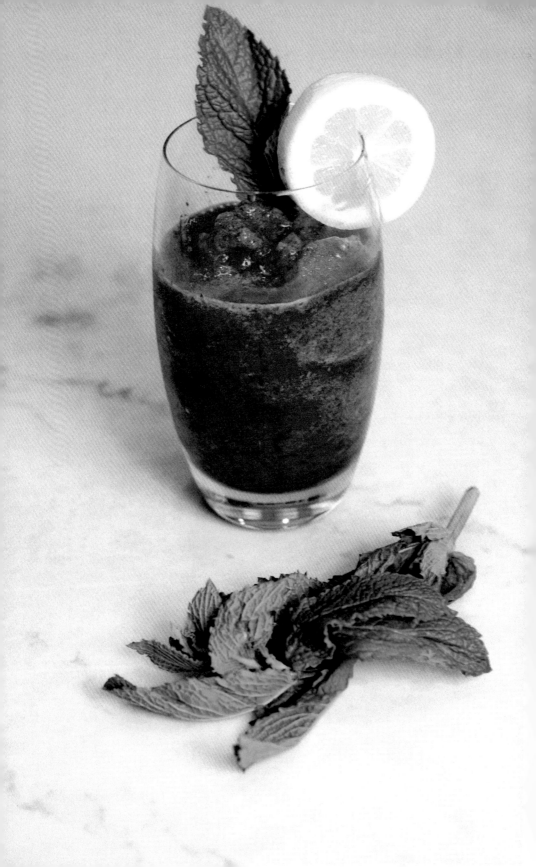

RASPBERRY LEMONADE CLEANSING SMOOTHIE

1 cup dandelion root tea
1 cup frozen raspberries
1 lemon
10 fresh mint leaves
1 TBSP raw local honey

Directions:
Blend until desired consistency is reached.

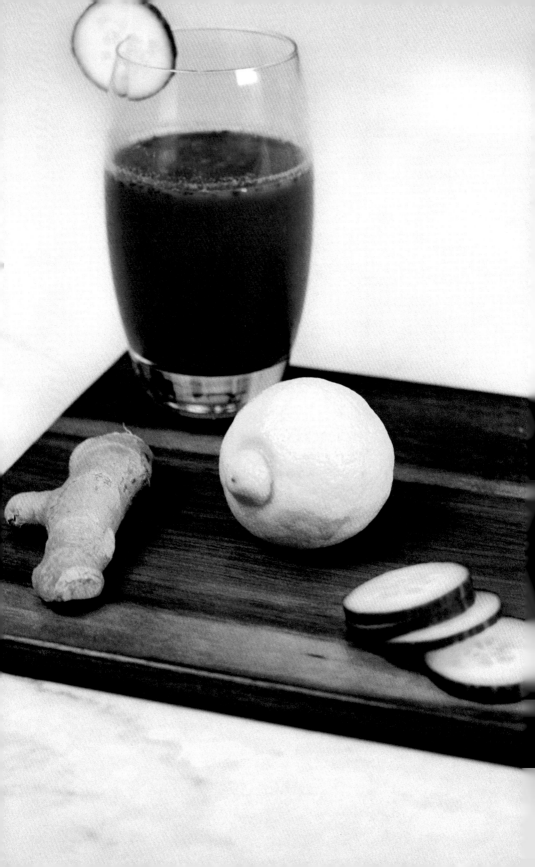

IMMUNITY JUICE

3 celery sticks
1 red apple (without the core)
1 inch ginger
1 cup parsley
1 cup spinach
1/2 cucumber
1/2 lemon

Directions:
Juice all ingredients.

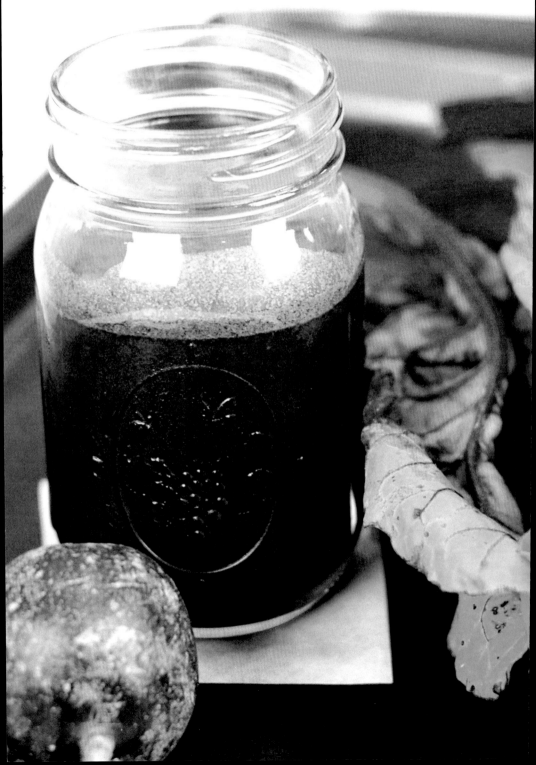

INTOXICATING DETOXIFICATION

1 cup of kale
2 leaves of Swiss chard
1 cup parsley
1/2 small beet
1/2 cup pineapple
2 medium green apples
1 sprig of fresh mint
1/2 lemon

Directions:
Juice all ingredients.

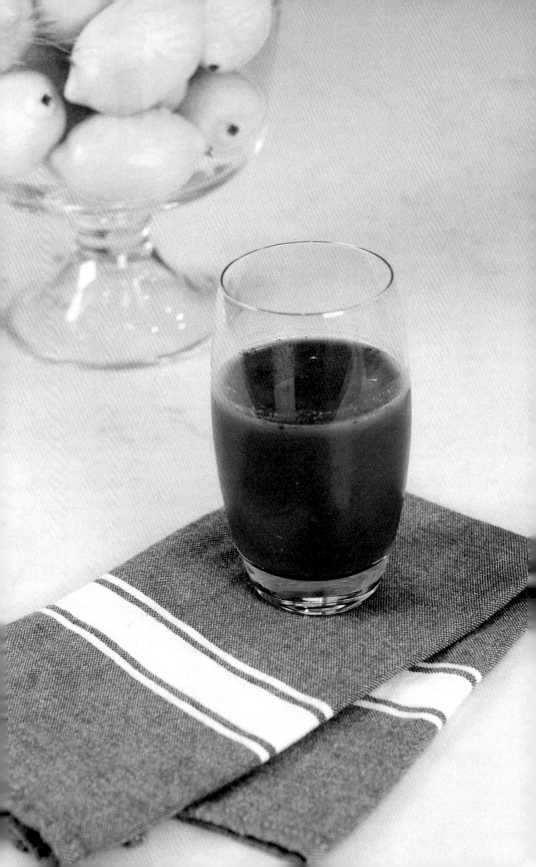

GREEN OBSESSION

1 heart of romaine lettuce
1 bag parsley (approx 2.5oz)
2 lemons
1 heart of celery
2 small green apples

Directions:
Juice all ingredients.

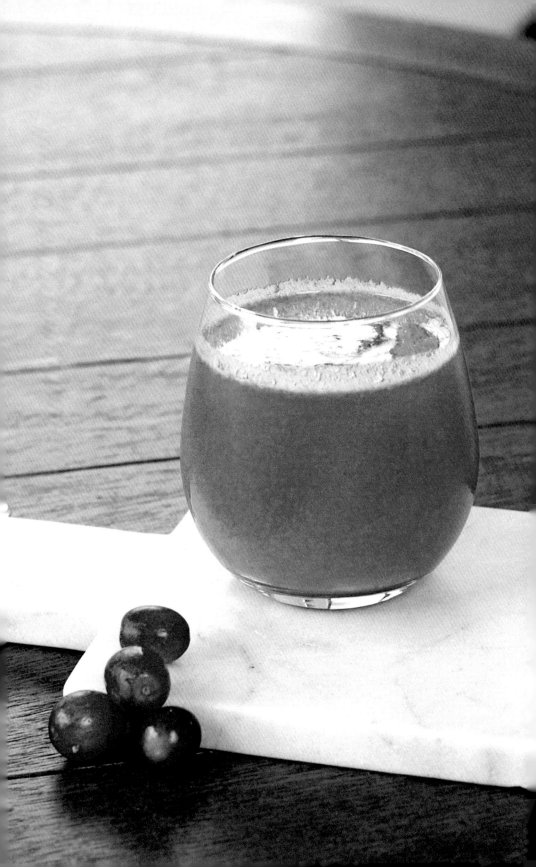

GRAPE CITRUS APPLE

2 cups red grapes
2 red apples (cored)
1 lemon

Directions:
Juice all ingredients.

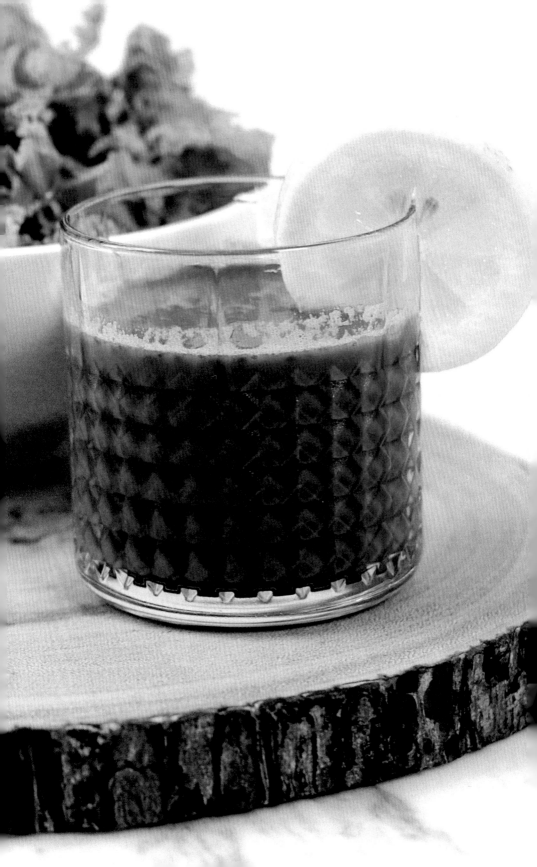

QUEEN OF GREEN

2 celery stalks
1 bag of parsley (approx. 2.5 oz)
2 cups spinach
1 lemon
4 kale leaves

Directions:
Juice all ingredients.

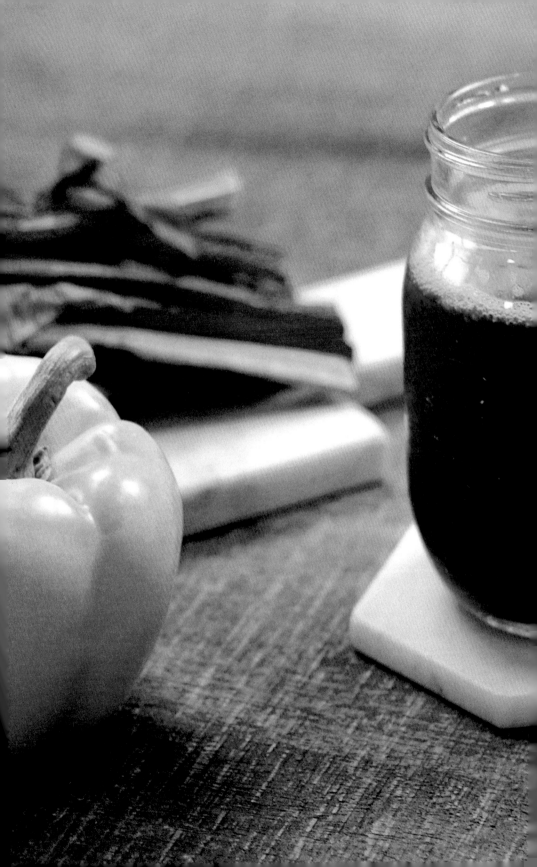

MEAN GREEN

8 broccoli spears
1 cup spinach
6 Swiss chard leaves
1 yellow bell pepper

Directions:
Juice all ingredients.

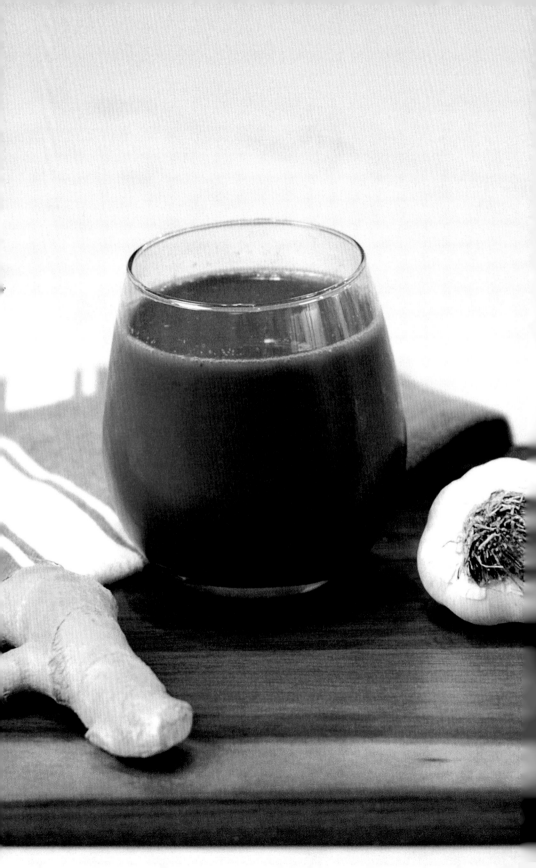

LEAN AND GREEN

4 leaves of romaine lettuce
2 cups spinach
8 broccoli spears
2 carrots
1 clove of garlic
1/2 inch ginger
1 lemon

Directions:
Juice all ingredients.

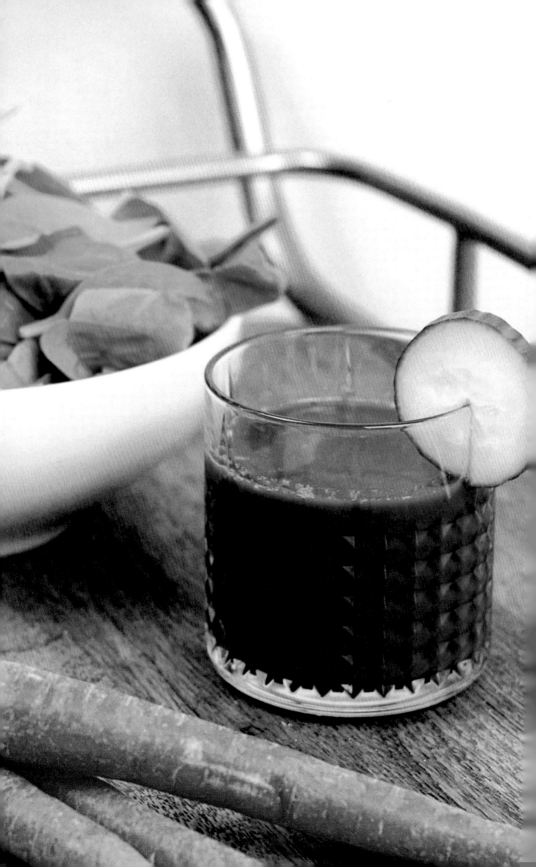

POPEYE'S BLEND

2 cups spinach
2 cucumbers
4 carrots

Directions:
Juice all ingredients.

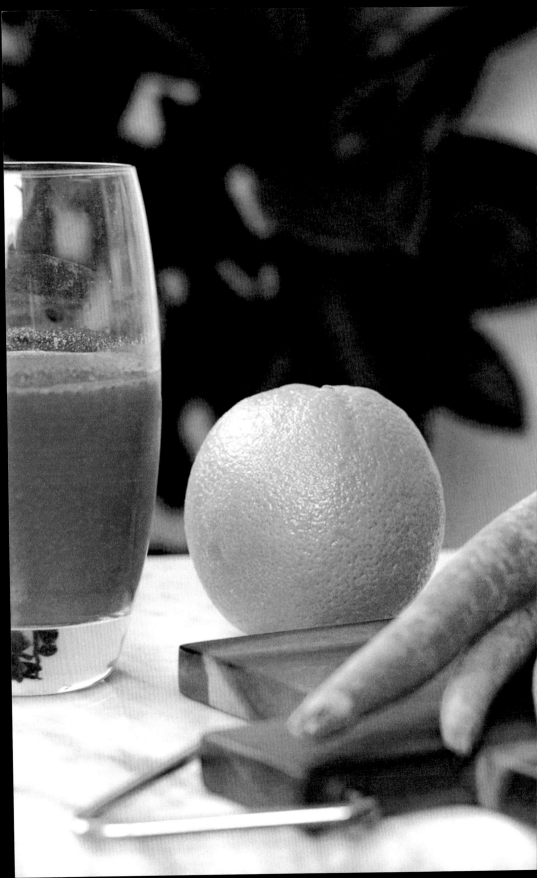

ORANGE CARROT JUICE

2 oranges
12 carrots

Directions:
Juice all ingredients.

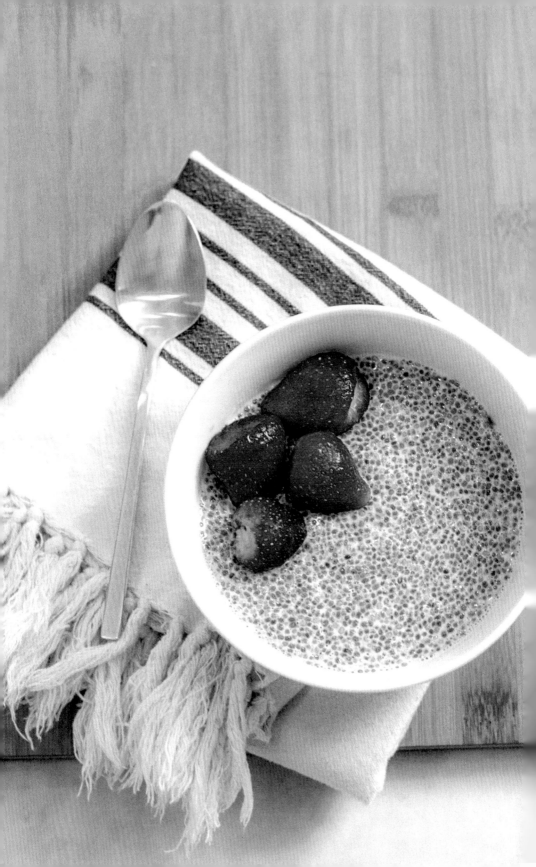

CHIA SEED PUDDING

1 cup vanilla-flavored unsweetened almond milk
1/4 cup chia seeds
1 cup strawberries
sprinkle of cinnamon

Directions:
In a medium bowl, gently whisk the almond milk and the chia seeds; let stand 30 minutes.

Stir to distribute the seeds if they have settled. Cover and refrigerate overnight.

The next day, top with strawberries and cinnamon.

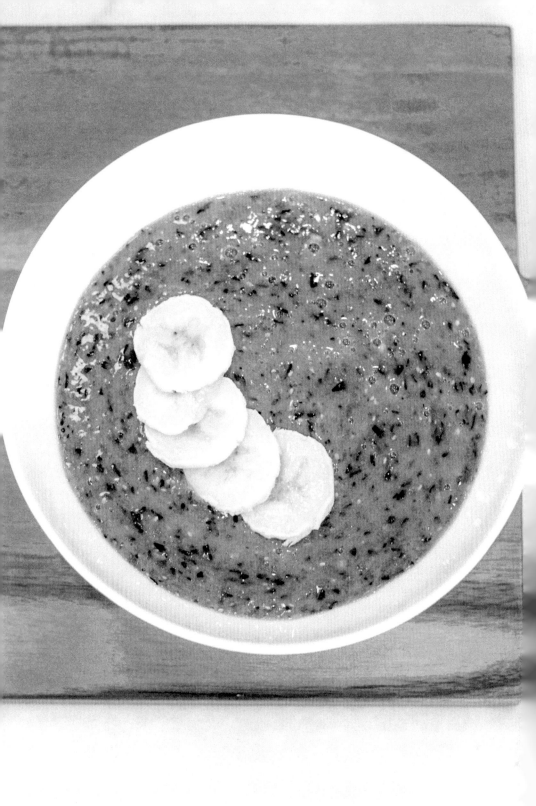

BLUEBERRY BANANA

2 cups blueberries
1 banana
2 TBSP chia seeds

Directions:
Blend and let sit for 5 minutes.

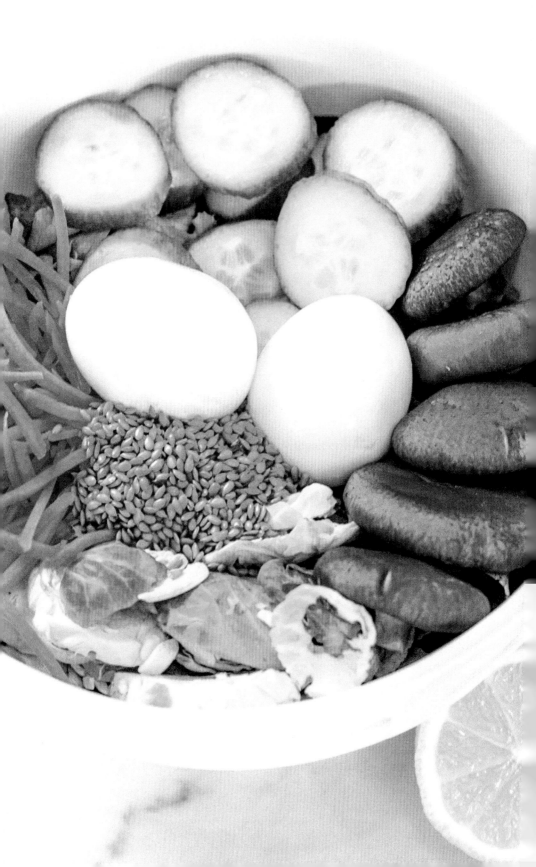

DETOX SALAD

2 cups organic mixed greens
1 cup Brussels sprouts (raw or sautéed)
1/2 cup organic shiitaki mushrooms (raw or sautéed)
1/3 cucumber (sliced)
1/2 cup shredded carrots
1 TBSP flaxseeds
2 hardboiled eggs

Dressing: 1 TBSP of extra virgin olive oil and the juice from 1 organic lemon

Directions:
Massage dressing on to greens, then top with vegetables.

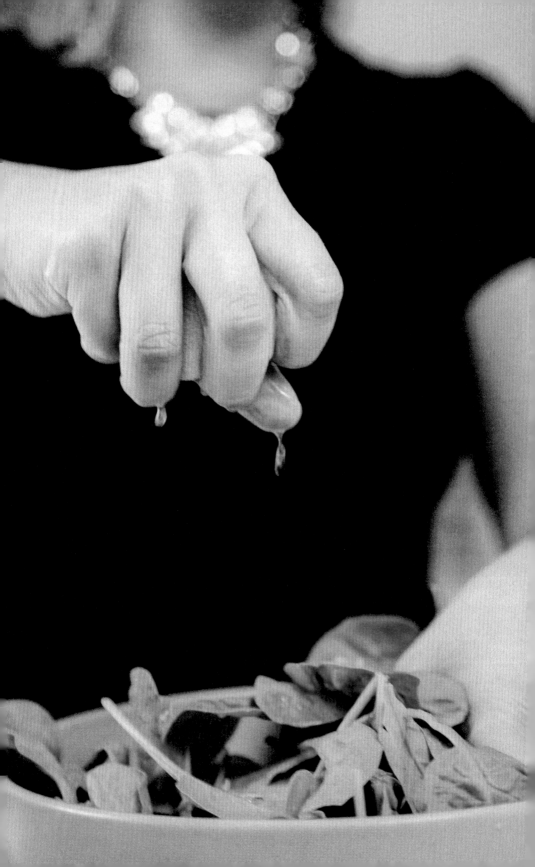

GROCERY SHOPPING LIST
We recommend that all ingredients are organic.

GREENS & VEGETABLES
3 heads of celery
6 inches of ginger root
3 bags of spinach
1 large bunch of parsley
1 large bunch of kale
1 large bunch of Swiss chard
1 large bunch of romaine lettuce
1 small beet
40 spears of broccoli
2 yellow bell peppers
7 cucumbers
53 large carrots
1 head of garlic
2 bags of mixed greens
3 cups of Brussels sprouts
2 cups of shiitake mushrooms

FRUIT
23 lemons
4 cups of frozen raspberries
2 bunches of fresh mint
9 red apples
6 green apples
1 pineapple
6 cups of red grapes
6 oranges
3 cups of strawberries
4 cups of blueberries
2 bananas

MISCELLANEOUS
1 package of dandelion root tea
1 package of parsley tea
1 package of green tea
1 jar of raw local honey
1 container of vanilla-flavored, unsweetened almond milk
1 package of chia seeds
1 package of flax seeds
6 eggs
1 bottle of extra virgin olive oil
1 bottle of Bragg's apple cider vinegar

GLOSSARY OF TERMS

ALKALINE
Any substance or food having a pH of 7 or more, basic, non-acidic. Dark leafy greens are an example of an alkaline food.

ANTIOXIDANTS
Antioxidants come from many of the fresh fruit and vegetables we eat on a daily basis. An antioxidant inhibits or even prevents oxidation, especially with stored food products and other molecules in the body. If these free radicals are left in the body, they can cause major problems and disease. Antioxidants are able to neutralize and eliminate free radicals before major damage occurs. Antioxidants can be found in goji berries, blueberries, dark chocolate, pecans, artichokes, and many other foods we consume daily.

FREE RADICALS
Free radicals are reactive atoms, or groups of atoms, that have at least one unpaired electron. Free radicals can be processed in the body, or brought in from outside sources, such as smoking, pollution, and other toxins. These free radicals damage our cells and have the ability to alter our DNA cell structure. The body has a built in defense for these free radicals, called antioxidants.

HEAVY METALS

Heavy metals are metallic chemical elements that are toxic or poisonous, even at low concentrations. A few examples of heavy metals are mercury, arsenic, chromium, and lead. They are found in food, water, air, and many common household items.

JUICE

A thin liquid made from fruits and vegetables, typically not containing any fiber, but is a rich source of vitamins and minerals. Easy for ones body to digest and absorb.

SMOOTHIE

Thick, pureed blend of fruit, vegetables, and liquid. Typically a good source of fiber, vitamins, and minerals. Many ingredients can be added to a smoothie, such as yogurt, milk, seeds, and protein powders to increase the protein, fiber, and fat content of the smoothie.

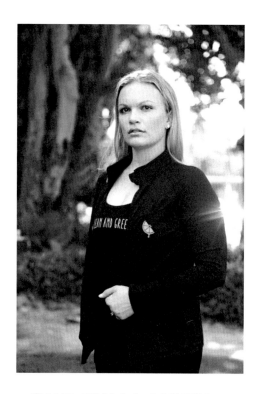

ONE FINAL NOTE...

We are given one body. Let's treat it with love, respect, and fuel our body with wholesome foods and ingredients that truly nourish us.

For more questions on health or wellness, contact Jennifer, jennifer@leanandgreenbody.com
or visit our website at
www.leanandgreenbody.com.

Be Well,

Jennifer

Made in the USA
Lexington, KY
11 January 2018